AGELESS VITALITY

(Unlocking the Secrets to Timeless Youth)

By

Dr. ROSE MYERS

Copyright@2023 Dr. Rose Myers

TABLE OF CONTENT

PREFACE

Welcome to "Ageless Vitality: Unlocking the Secrets to Timeless Youth." In a world where age is often associated with limitations and decline, this book sets out to challenge that notion. It invites you on a transformative journey to discover the secrets of maintaining a youthful age and embracing a vibrant, fulfilling life.

We live in an era where the desire to look and feel youthful has never been stronger. People are seeking ways to preserve their vitality, radiance, and zest for life, irrespective of their chronological age. The pursuit of youthfulness goes beyond mere aesthetics; it encompasses the physical, mental, and emotional aspects of our being.

In these pages, we delve into the art and science of maintaining a youthful age. We explore a holistic approach that encompasses nourishing our bodies with healthy habits, fostering a positive mindset, and cultivating habits that promote overall well-being.

Drawing from scientific research, ancient wisdom, and personal anecdotes, this book presents practical strategies, actionable advice, and inspiration to help you unlock your own fountain of youth.

However, it's essential to recognize that maintaining a youthful age is not about defying the natural process of aging. Instead, it's about embracing the beauty of each stage of life and nurturing our bodies, minds, and spirits to thrive at any age. The goal is to cultivate vitality, energy, and a genuine sense of joy that radiates from within.

Whether you are in your twenties, forties, or beyond, this book is for anyone who seeks to live with passion, purpose, and a youthful spirit. It is a guide to help you tap into your innate potential, make empowering choices, and create a life that exudes the vibrancy and wonder of youth.

So, let us embark on this trans-formative journey together. Get ready to discover the secrets, uncover your own path to ageless vitality, and embrace the joy of living a youthful life, regardless of the numbers on the calendar.

Remember, age is just a number, but the power to maintain a youthful age lies within you.

With excitement and anticipation, Dr.Rose Myers.

Chapter One

STAY ACTIVE

To stay active means to engage in regular physical activity and incorporate movement into your daily routine. Here's an explanation of what it means to stay active:

Engage in Regular Exercise: Incorporate a mix of cardiovascular exercises, such as brisk walking, jogging, or cycling, to keep your heart healthy and improve blood circulation. Aim for at least 150 minutes of moderate-intensity exercise per week.

Strength Training: Include strength training exercises like lifting weights, body-weight exercises, or resistance training. Building muscle helps improve posture, increase metabolism, and maintain a toned appearance.

Flexibility and Stretching: Incorporate stretching exercises and activities like yoga or Pilates to improve flexibility, prevent muscle stiffness, and maintain a youthful range of motion.

Stay Active Throughout the Day: Find opportunities to be active in your daily life. Take the stairs instead of the elevator, go for short walks during breaks, or engage in household chores that involve movement.

Try New Activities: Keep exercise exciting by trying different activities like dancing, swimming, hiking, or joining a sports club. Variety not only keeps you motivated but also engages different muscle groups.

Set Realistic Goals: Set achievable fitness goals that align with your abilities and interests. Start with small steps and gradually increase intensity and duration to avoid burnout or injuries.

Find a Workout Buddy: Partnering with a friend or family member can make exercise more enjoyable and help you stay motivated and accountable.

Mix Up Your Routine: Keep boredom at bay by varying your workouts. Try different exercise classes, outdoor activities, or online workout programs to keep your body challenged and engaged.

Listen to Your Body: Pay attention to any discomfort or pain during exercise. If something doesn't feel right, modify or consult a healthcare professional to prevent injuries and ensure safe and effective workouts.

Prioritize Active Hobbies: Incorporate physical activities you enjoy into your routine. Whether it's gardening, dancing, playing a sport, or walking your dog, finding joy in movement makes staying active sustainable and fun.

Be reminded that, staying active is not only about maintaining a youthful look but also about promoting overall health and well-being. Find activities that bring you joy, keep you motivated, and help you stay active for years to come.

Chapter Two

EAT BALANCED DIET

Eating a balanced diet means consuming a variety of foods that provide all the essential nutrients your body needs to function optimally. Here's an explanation of what it means to eat a balanced diet:

Essential Nutrients: A balanced diet provides a wide range of essential nutrients like vitamins, minerals, proteins, carbohydrates, and healthy fats. These nutrients support various bodily functions, promote healthy cell regeneration, and contribute to a youthful and vibrant appearance.

Skin Health: Certain nutrients, such as antioxidants, omega-3 fatty acids, and vitamins A, C, and E, play a crucial role in maintaining healthy skin. They help protect against oxidative stress, improve collagen production, and promote skin elasticity, reducing the appearance of wrinkles and fine lines.

Hydration: Many fruits and vegetables are high in water content, helping to keep your body hydrated. Well-hydrated skin appears plump, smooth, and youthful, while dehydration can lead to dryness and premature aging.

Collagen Formation: Protein-rich foods, like lean meats, fish, legumes, and dairy products, provide amino acids necessary for collagen production. Collagen is a structural protein that keeps the skin firm, elastic, and youthful-looking.

Antioxidant Protection: Fruits and vegetables are rich in antioxidants that help combat free radicals, unstable molecules that can damage cells and contribute to aging. Consuming a variety of colorful fruits and veggies provides a broad spectrum of antioxidants to support overall health and maintain a youthful glow.

Energy and Vitality: A balanced diet provides the necessary energy to fuel your body and keep you active and vibrant. It ensures you have the stamina and vitality to engage in physical activities, maintain muscle mass, and enjoy a youthful lifestyle.

Bone Health: Adequate intake of calcium, vitamin D, and other bone-supporting nutrients is essential for maintaining strong and healthy bones. A balanced diet that includes dairy products, leafy greens, nuts, and fortified foods helps reduce the risk of osteoporosis and supports overall skeletal health.

Healthy Weight Management: A balanced diet promotes healthy weight maintenance or weight loss if needed. Excess weight can contribute to various health issues and accelerate the aging process. By nourishing your body with the right balance of nutrients, you support a healthy metabolism and prevent the negative effects of weight gain.

Mental Well-being: Proper nutrition plays a significant role in maintaining mental clarity and emotional well-being. Consuming a balanced diet that includes omega-3 fatty acids, B vitamins, and other nutrients supports brain health and helps reduce the risk of cognitive decline, promoting a youthful state of mind.

Disease Prevention: A balanced diet rich in fruits, vegetables, whole grains, and lean proteins helps protect against chronic diseases such as heart disease, diabetes, and certain cancers. By preventing or managing these conditions, you promote overall health and longevity, contributing to a youthful age.

Recall that, a balanced diet is not just about individual foods but about the overall pattern of your eating habits. Embrace variety, moderation, and mindful eating to nourish your body, support your well-being, and maintain a youthful age inside and out

Chapter Three

HYDRATE

To hydrate means to provide your body with an adequate amount of fluids, typically water, to maintain proper hydration levels. Here's an explanation of how hydration contribute to youthful age:

Skin Moisture: Adequate hydration helps keep your skin moisturized from within. It promotes a healthy skin barrier function, preventing dryness, flakiness, and dullness. Well-hydrated skin appears plump, smooth, and youthful.

Wrinkle Reduction: Proper hydration helps reduce the appearance of wrinkles and fine lines. When your body is well-hydrated, your skin maintains its elasticity, making it less prone to developing premature wrinkles and maintaining a youthful look.

Skin Elasticity: Water is essential for maintaining skin elasticity. It keeps your skin cells plump and supports the production of collagen and elastin, two proteins that contribute to skin's firmness and youthful bounce.

Skin Tone and Radiance: Hydrated skin has a more even tone and radiant appearance. When you're well-hydrated, your skin reflects light better, giving it a healthy glow and minimizing the appearance of dullness or sallowness.

Nutrient Transport: Proper hydration ensures the efficient transport of nutrients to your skin cells. It helps deliver essential vitamins, minerals, and antioxidants that support overall skin health and provide a youthful appearance.

Toxin Removal: Staying hydrated supports the removal of toxins and waste products from your body, including those that can affect your skin's health and appearance. Proper hydration helps flush out impurities, promoting clearer and healthier skin.

Prevents Dryness and Itchiness: Dehydration can lead to dry, itchy, and irritated skin. By maintaining adequate hydration, you help prevent these uncomfortable skin conditions and maintain a soft, supple, and youthful skin texture.

Reduces Puffiness: Dehydration can contribute to puffiness and under-eye bags. Proper hydration helps flush out excess fluid and reduces the appearance of puffiness, leaving your face looking more youthful and refreshed.

Hair and Nail Health: Hydration is not only important for your skin but also for your hair and nails. Well-hydrated hair is more lustrous and less prone to breakage, while hydrated nails are stronger and less brittle, contributing to an overall youthful appearance.

General Well-being: Staying hydrated promotes overall well-being, which reflects in your appearance. When you're properly hydrated, you feel more energized, vibrant, and youthful, radiating a healthy and youthful aura.

Always remember, maintaining hydration is not only about drinking water but also about incorporating hydrating foods, such as fruits and vegetables, into your diet. Pay attention to your body's signals and aim to drink water throughout the day to maintain proper hydration levels and support a youthful age.

Chapter Four

PROTECT YOUR SKIN

Skin protection refers to the practices and measures taken to safeguard the health and well-being of your skin. Here's an explanation of how skin protection contributes to youthful age:

Sun Damage Prevention: Protecting your skin from the harmful effects of the sun is vital for maintaining a youthful appearance. Prolonged sun exposure can lead to premature aging signs like wrinkles, fine lines, age spots, and sagging skin.

UV Radiation Protection: Shielding your skin from UV radiation helps prevent damage to the collagen and elastin fibers that give your skin its elasticity and firmness. By minimizing UV exposure, you reduce the risk of developing sunburns, skin discoloration, and photo-aging.

Wrinkle Reduction: Sun protection plays a significant role in reducing the formation of wrinkles and fine lines. UV rays can break down collagen and elastin, resulting in skin that appears aged and less smooth. Consistently protecting your skin from the sun helps maintain its youthful elasticity and minimizes the appearance of wrinkles.

Skin Cancer Prevention: By protecting your skin from harmful UV radiation, you decrease the risk of developing skin cancer. Skin cancer is a serious health concern that can not only impact your physical well-being but also contribute to premature aging.

Even Skin Tone: Consistent sun protection helps maintain an even skin tone by preventing the formation of dark spots and hyper-pigmentation caused by sun damage. This promotes a youthful and radiant complexion.

Moisture Retention: Protecting your skin helps retain moisture, preventing dehydration and dryness. Dry skin can appear dull, rough, and aged, while well-moisturized skin maintains a healthy and youthful glow.

Barrier Function Maintenance: External aggressors like pollution, wind, and harsh weather conditions can damage your skin's protective barrier. By using appropriate skincare products and protective measures, you help maintain the integrity of your skin's barrier, reducing the risk of moisture loss and maintaining a youthful complexion.

Early Aging Prevention: Skin protection helps prevent early signs of aging. By minimizing exposure to environmental factors and using suitable skincare products, you preserve the health and vitality of your skin, promoting a youthful appearance for longer.

Skincare Product Effectiveness: Protecting your skin enhances the effectiveness of your skincare routine. When your skin is shielded from external aggressors, it allows your skincare products to work more efficiently, providing maximum benefits for maintaining a youthful age.

Self-Care and Long-Term Well-being: Prioritizing skin protection is a form of self-care that contributes to your long-term well-being. By showing care and concern for your skin's health, you cultivate healthy habits that support a youthful mindset and lifestyle.

Remember, protecting your skin goes beyond just using sunscreen. It also involves seeking shade when the sun is strongest, wearing protective clothing, using hats and sunglasses, and adopting a comprehensive skincare routine that includes cleansing, moisturizing, and incorporating suitable products for your skin type. By making skin protection a habit, you can enjoy a youthful and healthy complexion for years to come.

Chapter Five

GET ENOUGH SLEEP

Getting enough sleep means giving your body and mind the rest they need to function optimally. Here's an explanation of how getting enough sleep contributes to youthful age:

Skin Repair and Regeneration: During sleep, your body undergoes crucial repair processes, including the regeneration of skin cells. Sufficient sleep allows your skin to recover from daily environmental stressors, promoting a healthy complexion and a youthful appearance.

Collagen Production: Sleep plays a vital role in collagen production, a protein that gives your skin its strength and elasticity. Ample sleep helps maintain optimal collagen levels, reducing the appearance of wrinkles and fine lines and keeping your skin looking youthful and supple.

Dark Circle Reduction: Lack of sleep can contribute to the formation of dark circles and under-eye bags. Sufficient sleep allows the delicate skin around your eyes to rejuvenate, minimizing the appearance of puffiness and dark circles, promoting a fresh and youthful look.

Improved Skin Tone: A good night's sleep contributes to a more even and vibrant skin tone. When you're well-rested, your skin appears brighter, healthier, and free from dullness or sallowness, promoting a youthful complexion.

Hormonal Balance: Adequate sleep helps regulate hormones, including those involved in the aging process. Hormonal imbalances can accelerate aging and affect the health and appearance of your skin. Restful sleep supports hormonal balance, promoting a youthful and radiant look.

Reduced Inflammation: Lack of sleep can lead to increased inflammation in the body, which can contribute to skin issues like acne, redness, and irritation. Sufficient sleep helps reduce inflammation, promoting a calm and healthy complexion.

Increased Blood Circulation: Quality sleep enhances blood circulation, delivering essential nutrients and oxygen to your skin cells. This nourishment supports optimal skin health, promoting a youthful and glowing appearance.

Stress Reduction: Adequate sleep helps manage stress levels, which can impact your skin's health and aging process. Chronic stress can lead to the release of stress hormones that contribute to premature aging. By getting enough sleep, you reduce stress and support a more youthful and relaxed appearance.

Eye Health: Restful sleep is essential for maintaining healthy eyes. It helps prevent eye fatigue, puffiness, and dryness, reducing the appearance of tired-looking eyes and promoting a youthful gaze.

Overall Well-being: Sufficient sleep is vital for your overall well-being, and a rested mind and body reflect in your appearance. When you're well-rested, you have more energy, vitality, and a positive mindset, contributing to a youthful and vibrant aura.

Recall, prioritizing quality sleep involves establishing a consistent sleep routine, creating a sleep-friendly environment, and adopting relaxation techniques before bed. By making adequate sleep a priority, you can support a youthful age and enjoy the benefits of a well-rested mind and body.

Chapter Six

MANAGE STRESS

Managing stress is all about finding ways to deal with it and keep yourself cool, calm, and collected. Here's an explanation of how managing stress promotes youthful age:

Reduced Premature Aging: Chronic stress can accelerate the aging process, leading to the formation of wrinkles, fine lines, and dull skin. By managing stress, you minimize its negative impact on your skin, helping to maintain a youthful and radiant complexion.

Skin Health: Stress can worsen skin conditions such as acne, eczema, and psoriasis. Effective stress management techniques, such as relaxation exercises and mindfulness, help reduce flare-ups and promote healthier-looking skin.

Collagen Preservation: High levels of stress can break down collagen, the protein responsible for maintaining skin's elasticity and firmness. By managing stress, you support collagen preservation, reducing the appearance of sagging skin and maintaining a more youthful look.

Skin Radiance: Stress can lead to dull, lackluster skin. By effectively managing stress, you enhance blood circulation, allowing for better nutrient and oxygen delivery to your skin cells. This promotes a natural glow and a more youthful and vibrant complexion.

Reduced Eye Fatigue: Stress can contribute to eye strain, puffiness, and dark circles. Through stress management techniques like relaxation and adequate sleep, you minimize the impact of stress on your eyes, promoting a refreshed and youthful appearance.

Hair Health: Stress can lead to hair loss, thinning, and a dull appearance. By managing stress, you help maintain healthy hair growth and prevent premature aging of your hair, promoting a more youthful and vibrant mane.

Muscle Tension Reduction: Stress often manifests as muscle tension and tightness, especially in the face and neck areas. By practicing stress management techniques such as deep breathing and stretching exercises, you relax your facial muscles, reducing the formation of tension lines and promoting a more youthful facial expression.

Improved Sleep Quality: Stress can disrupt sleep patterns, leading to sleep deprivation and fatigue. By effectively managing stress, you improve sleep quality, allowing for optimal skin repair and regeneration during the night, resulting in a more youthful appearance.

Mental Well-being: Stress management is crucial for maintaining a positive mindset and overall mental well-being. When you're less stressed, you feel happier, more confident, and youthful, which reflects in your demeanor and appearance.

Overall Health Promotion: Chronic stress can have detrimental effects on your overall health, including cardiovascular issues, weakened immune system, and chronic conditions. By managing stress, you promote overall well-being, contributing to a healthier and more youthful age.

Remember, effective stress management involves finding techniques that work for you, such as exercise, meditation, hobbies, or seeking support from friends, family, or professionals. By prioritizing stress management, you can maintain a youthful age and enjoy the benefits of a calmer and more vibrant lifestyle

Chapter Seven

STAY SOCIALLY CONNECTED

Staying socially connected is essential for promoting a youthful age. Here's a brief explanation of how social connections contribute to a youthful appearance:

Mental Stimulation: Engaging in social interactions provides mental stimulation, which keeps your mind active and sharp. It helps prevent cognitive decline and supports a youthful and agile mindset.

Emotional Well-being: Social connections foster a sense of belonging, support, and happiness. When you have strong social ties, you experience positive emotions, reducing stress and promoting a youthful and vibrant outlook on life.

Stress Reduction: Social support acts as a buffer against stress. By having a network of friends and loved ones, you have people to turn to during challenging times, which helps reduce stress levels. Lower stress levels contribute to a more youthful appearance.

Self-Care Accountability: Being socially connected often involves participating in activities with others. This can include exercise, healthy eating, and self-care practices. Social connections provide accountability and motivation, promoting healthy habits that contribute to a youthful lifestyle.

Increased Physical Activity: Social connections often involve engaging in group activities or sports, which encourage physical movement and exercise. Regular physical activity supports cardiovascular health, muscle tone, and overall vitality, contributing to a youthful age.

Intellectual Growth: Social interactions expose you to diverse perspectives and ideas, fostering intellectual growth and curiosity. Engaging in stimulating conversations and sharing experiences with others keeps your mind active and promotes a youthful and inquisitive mindset.

Confidence Boost: Positive social connections boost self-confidence and self-esteem. When you feel supported and valued by others, it reflects in your posture, demeanor, and overall appearance, contributing to a youthful and radiant presence.

Sense of Purpose: Social connections provide a sense of purpose and meaning. By engaging in social activities and forming meaningful relationships, you feel a greater sense of fulfillment and purpose in life, which positively impacts your overall well-being and youthful mindset.

Laughter and Joy: Social interactions often involve laughter and enjoyment. Laughing and experiencing joy release endorphins, which are natural mood enhancers. Regular moments of laughter contribute to a more youthful and joyful demeanor.

Positive Energy: Being socially connected exposes you to positive energy from others. Surrounding yourself with uplifting and supportive individuals helps create a positive atmosphere, promoting a youthful and vibrant aura.

Be reminded that, staying socially connected involves nurturing existing relationships and actively seeking opportunities to meet new people. Join clubs, participate in community events, and maintain regular communication with friends and family. By prioritizing social connections, you can promote a youthful age and enjoy the benefits of a rich and fulfilling social life.

Chapter Eight

PROTECT YOUR EYES

Protecting your eyes is important for promoting a youthful age. Here's a brief explanation of how eye protection contributes to a youthful appearance:

Preventing Wrinkles: Protecting your eyes from harmful UV radiation and squinting helps prevent the formation of wrinkles around the eyes, known as crow's feet. UV rays and repetitive facial expressions can accelerate the development of fine lines, so using sunglasses and avoiding excessive squinting supports a more youthful appearance.

Dark Circle Reduction: Proper eye protection can help reduce the appearance of dark circles under the eyes. Dark circles can make you appear tired and older. By protecting your eyes from factors like lack of sleep, allergies, and sun damage, you can minimize the occurrence of dark circles, promoting a fresh and youthful look.

Minimizing Eye Strain: Protecting your eyes from digital eye strain and excessive screen time can prevent eye fatigue, dryness, and redness. By giving your eyes regular breaks, using proper lighting, and maintaining a comfortable distance from screens, you reduce the risk of strained, tired-looking eyes, contributing to a more youthful appearance.

Eye Health Preservation: Protecting your eyes from environmental factors and potential injuries helps preserve their long-term health. By wearing appropriate eye protection during activities such as sports, DIY projects, and outdoor work, you reduce the risk of eye injuries that could lead to long-term complications and affect your overall youthful age.

Maintaining Clear Vision: Regular eye check-ups and proper eyewear contribute to maintaining clear and sharp vision. Good vision enhances your overall appearance and allows you to see the world in its full clarity, promoting a youthful and engaged perspective.

Prevention of Eye Diseases: Eye protection measures, such as wearing sunglasses that block harmful UV rays, help reduce the risk of developing eye diseases like cataracts and age-related macular degeneration. By safeguarding your eyes from harmful UV radiation, you promote long-term eye health and maintain a youthful vision.

Reducing Puffiness and Under-Eye Bags: Eye protection, including proper sleep and hydration, can help reduce puffiness and under-eye bags. By taking care of your overall health and practicing good sleep habits, you minimize fluid retention and inflammation around the eyes, promoting a youthful and well-rested appearance.

Preserving Eye Sparkle: Protecting your eyes from excessive exposure to dry environments, pollution, and harsh chemicals helps maintain their natural sparkle and brightness. By avoiding irritants and maintaining good eye hygiene, you promote vibrant and youthful-looking eyes.

Promoting Confidence: Taking care of your eyes and protecting them from potential harm boosts your confidence and self-esteem. Feeling confident in your eye health and appearance contributes to a more youthful and positive outlook.

Overall Facial Harmony: The eyes play a significant role in facial aesthetics. By protecting your eyes and maintaining their health, you contribute to overall facial harmony and a youthful appearance. Healthy, bright eyes are a key element in looking vibrant and youthful.

Remember, eye protection involves various measures, such as wearing sunglasses with UV protection, using proper eye safety gear, practicing good eye hygiene, and seeking regular eye check-ups. By prioritizing eye protection, you can maintain a youthful age and enjoy the benefits of healthy, vibrant eyes.

Chapter Nine

PRACTICE SKINCARE

Practicing skincare is crucial for promoting a youthful age. Here's a brief explanation of how skincare promotes a youthful appearance:

Moisture and Hydration: Skincare routines often involve using moisturizers and hydrating products. These help nourish the skin, maintain its moisture barrier, and prevent dryness. Well-hydrated skin appears plump, supple, and youthful.

Wrinkle Prevention: Skincare products, such as serums and creams with anti-aging ingredients like retinol and peptides, can help minimize the appearance of wrinkles and fine lines. Regular use of these products supports collagen production and improves skin elasticity, promoting a smoother and more youthful complexion.

Sun Protection: Sunscreen is a crucial part of skincare. By protecting your skin from harmful UV radiation, you reduce the risk of premature aging, such as wrinkles, age spots, and sagging skin. Sun protection is essential for maintaining a youthful appearance and preventing long-term damage.

Even Skin Tone: Skincare routines often include products that target hyper-pigmentation, such as dark spots and uneven skin tone. By using ingredients like vitamin C and niacinamide, you can promote a more even complexion and a youthful, radiant glow.

Skin Renewal: Exfoliation is an important step in skincare. It helps remove dead skin cells, revealing fresh, new skin underneath. Regular exfoliation promotes skin renewal, enhances texture, and encourages a youthful and smoother appearance.

Reducing Puffiness and Dark Circles: Skincare products like eye creams and serums can help reduce under-eye puffiness and the appearance of dark circles.

These products often contain ingredients that hydrate and soothe the delicate skin around the eyes, promoting a more rested and youthful look.

Acne Prevention and Treatment: Skincare routines can address acne concerns, helping to prevent breakouts and minimize the appearance of acne scars. By using products with acne-fighting ingredients like salicylic acid or benzoyl peroxide, you can promote clearer, healthier-looking skin and a more youthful complexion.

Boosting Skin Radiance: Skincare products that contain antioxidants, such as vitamin E and green tea extract, help fight free radicals and environmental damage. By incorporating these products into your routine, you can enhance your skin's radiance, promoting a youthful and vibrant glow.

Skin Protection: Skincare routines often involve using products that act as a protective barrier against environmental pollutants and irritants. By shielding your skin from these external factors, you minimize their damaging effects and maintain a healthier and more youthful appearance.

Self-Care and Confidence: Practicing skincare can be a form of self-care, providing time for relaxation and pampering. Taking care of your skin and investing in skincare products can boost your confidence, leading to a more positive mindset and a youthful aura.

Remember, establishing a consistent skincare routine tailored to your skin type and concerns is key. This may involve cleansing, moisturizing, using targeted treatments, and wearing sunscreen daily. By prioritizing skincare, you can promote a youthful age and enjoy the benefits of healthy, radiant skin.

Chapter Ten

MAINTAIN GOOD POSTURE

Maintaining good posture plays a significant role in promoting a youthful age. Here's a brief explanation of how good posture contributes to a youthful appearance:

Alignment and Balance: Good posture helps align your body properly, distributing weight evenly across your muscles and joints. This balanced alignment reduces the strain on specific areas and promotes overall body symmetry, contributing to a more youthful and attractive physique.

Muscle Tone and Strength: Maintaining good posture requires engaging your core muscles, including the abdominal and back muscles. Regularly activating these muscles through good posture helps strengthen them, leading to improved muscle tone and a more youthful-looking body.

Spinal Health: Good posture supports the natural curvature of the spine, preventing excessive strain on the spinal discs, vertebrae, and nerves. By maintaining proper alignment, you reduce the risk of developing spinal problems that can affect your posture and contribute to an aged appearance.

Confidence and Presence: Standing tall with good posture exudes confidence and presence. It creates a positive impression and projects a youthful, vibrant energy to others. Good posture enhances your overall presence and boosts self-esteem, making you feel and appear more youthful.

Respiratory Function: Proper posture allows your lungs to fully expand and your diaphragm to function efficiently. This promotes optimal oxygen intake and circulation, supporting overall vitality and a youthful glow.

Digestive Health: Good posture helps maintain proper organ alignment and encourages healthy digestion. When your body is properly aligned, it promotes optimal digestion and absorption of nutrients, leading to improved overall health and a more youthful appearance.

Joint Health: Good posture reduces stress on the joints, minimizing the risk of joint pain, stiffness, and age-related conditions like arthritis. By preserving joint health through proper alignment, you can maintain mobility and a youthful range of motion.

Facial Appearance: Slouching or poor posture can contribute to sagging skin and a less defined jawline. Maintaining good posture keeps the head lifted and helps prevent the appearance of a double chin or jowls, promoting a more youthful facial structure.

Body Language: Good posture enhances your body language, making you appear more open, approachable, and confident. It positively influences how others perceive you and contributes to a youthful and vibrant presence.

Long-Term Health Benefits: Consistently practicing good posture not only promotes a youthful appearance but also contributes to long-term health. By reducing the risk of musculoskeletal problems, improving circulation, and supporting optimal organ function, good posture helps you age gracefully and maintain a youthful body.

Have in mind that, maintaining good posture involves being mindful of your alignment while sitting, standing, and moving. Regular exercise, stretching, and core-strengthening activities can also help improve posture. By prioritizing good posture, you can enjoy the benefits of a more youthful, confident, and healthy physical presence.

Chapter Eleven

CHALLENGE YOUR MIND

Challenging your mind is an essential factor in promoting a youthful age. Here's a brief explanation of how mental stimulation contributes to a youthful mindset and appearance:

Cognitive Agility: Engaging in mentally challenging activities such as puzzles, games, or learning new skills keeps your mind sharp and agile. It stimulates neural connections and promotes cognitive flexibility, allowing you to adapt to new situations and challenges with ease, which is a characteristic of a youthful mindset.

Memory Enhancement: Keeping your mind active and engaged through mental challenges helps improve memory retention and recall. By exercising your memory regularly, you can maintain a sharp and youthful memory capacity.

Creativity and Innovation: Challenging your mind encourages creativity and fosters innovative thinking. It allows you to explore new ideas, problem-solving strategies, and alternative perspectives, which are vital for maintaining a youthful, adaptable, and forward-thinking mindset.

Emotional Resilience: Mental stimulation helps build emotional resilience by enhancing your ability to cope with stress, setbacks, and changes. A resilient mindset promotes a positive outlook, reducing the impact of negative emotions and contributing to a more youthful and vibrant demeanor.

Lifelong Learning: Actively seeking new knowledge and learning experiences keeps your mind curious, engaged, and open to growth. Lifelong learning contributes to personal development, expanding your horizons and keeping you youthful in your thirst for knowledge.

Confidence and Self-Esteem: Challenging your mind and achieving mental milestones boosts confidence and self-esteem. Accomplishing intellectual challenges, whether big or small, reinforces a sense of capability and contributes to a youthful, self-assured demeanor.

Brain Health: Engaging in mentally stimulating activities supports overall brain health and can help reduce the risk of age-related cognitive decline. By challenging your mind, you promote longevity and maintain cognitive vitality, contributing to a youthful age.

Social Engagement: Many mentally stimulating activities involve social interaction, such as group discussions or participating in team-based challenges. Social engagement provides mental stimulation, fosters connection, and contributes to a youthful, socially vibrant lifestyle.

Problem-Solving Skills: Challenging your mind sharpens your problem-solving abilities. It improves your analytical thinking, decision-making skills, and adaptability, which are crucial for navigating the complexities of life with a youthful and resilient mindset.

Quality of Life: Mental stimulation enhances overall quality of life, promoting a sense of purpose, fulfillment, and satisfaction. It keeps you mentally active, engaged, and motivated, allowing you to embrace life's challenges and opportunities with a youthful and enthusiastic approach.

To promote a youthful age through mental stimulation, incorporate activities such as reading, learning new hobbies, playing brain games, engaging in creative pursuits, or pursuing higher education. By challenging your mind and embracing a lifelong pursuit of knowledge and growth, you can maintain a youthful mindset and enjoy the benefits of mental vitality.

Chapter Twelve

LAUGH AND HAVE FUN

Laughing and having fun mean engaging in activities and experiences that bring joy, amusement, and a sense of enjoyment. Laughing and having fun play a significant role in promoting a youthful age. Here's a casual explanation of how they contribute to maintaining a youthful outlook:

Joyful Medicine: Laughing and having fun release endorphins, which are feel-good hormones that can improve your mood and overall well-being. When you engage in activities that bring you joy and make you laugh, it creates a positive state of mind that can make you feel more youthful and vibrant.

Stress Buster: Laughter and fun activities help reduce stress levels. They act as a natural stress reliever, helping to alleviate tension, anxiety, and worries. By managing stress, you can prevent its negative impact on your physical and mental health, contributing to a more youthful appearance and outlook.

Energy Booster: Laughing and having fun can increase your energy levels. When you engage in activities that bring you joy, it boosts your vitality and enthusiasm, making you feel more energized and youthful.

Social Connection: Laughing and having fun often occur in social settings, allowing you to connect with others and build relationships. Social connections are essential for a sense of belonging and happiness, which can contribute to a more positive and youthful mindset.

Youthful Perspective: Laughing and having fun help you maintain a lighthearted and playful perspective on life. They remind you not to take things too seriously and to find joy in the simplest moments. This youthful mindset can positively impact your overall outlook and attitude.

Inner Child Rediscovery: Engaging in activities that make you laugh and have fun can tap into your inner child. It allows you to embrace spontaneity, curiosity, and a sense of wonder, which are often associated with youthfulness.

Positive Vibes: Laughter and fun create a positive atmosphere and can influence the people around you. When you radiate positivity, it can enhance your relationships and interactions, making you appear more youthful and approachable.

E***motional Well-being:*** Laughing and having fun contribute to emotional well-being. They can enhance your resilience, optimism, and ability to cope with challenges, which are important aspects of maintaining a youthful spirit.

Mental Agility: Engaging in fun activities, games, and humor exercises can stimulate your brain and promote mental agility. It keeps your mind active, sharp, and adaptable, contributing to a more youthful cognitive function.

Wrinkle Eraser: Believe it or not, laughter can even have physical benefits. When you laugh, it engages multiple facial muscles, which can help tone and tighten the skin temporarily. So, laughing and having fun may give you a natural "face-lift" and a more youthful appearance.

Always remember, incorporating laughter and fun into your life is about finding activities and experiences that genuinely make you happy. Surround yourself with people who bring joy and embrace opportunities to laugh and have fun. It's an enjoyable way to stay youthful, both in mind and spirit!

Chapter Thirteen

PRACTICE GRATITUDE

Practicing gratitude can contribute to maintaining a youthful age by fostering a positive mindset and outlook on life. Here's an explanation of how gratitude promotes a youthful age:

Attitude of Appreciation: Practicing gratitude involves recognizing and appreciating the good things in your life, both big and small. It's like having a grateful heart that focuses on the positives rather than dwelling on the negatives.

Positive Perspective: Gratitude helps shift your perspective towards the positive aspects of life. By acknowledging and being thankful for what you have, you cultivate a more optimistic and hopeful outlook, which can make you feel more youthful and energized.

Stress Reduction: Gratitude acts as a natural stress reliever. When you focus on the things you're grateful for, it can help reduce anxiety, worries, and negative emotions, promoting a sense of calmness and inner peace. Managing stress positively contributes to a youthful appearance and overall well-being.

Improved Relationships: Expressing gratitude towards others strengthens your relationships and fosters a sense of connection. When you appreciate and acknowledge the people in your life, it can deepen your bonds, creating a positive and supportive social network that contributes to a more youthful and vibrant life.

Mindfulness and Presence: Practicing gratitude encourages you to be present in the moment and mindful of the blessings around you. It helps you slow down, savor the little joys, and fully experience life's wonders, promoting a sense of wonder and curiosity often associated with youthfulness.

Emotional Well-being: Gratitude positively impacts your emotional well-being. It increases feelings of happiness, contentment, and fulfillment. When you nurture positive emotions through gratitude, it can enhance your overall mood and mental well-being, reflecting a youthful and vibrant spirit.

Resilience Booster: Gratitude cultivates resilience and the ability to bounce back from challenges. By focusing on what you're grateful for, you build a sense of inner strength and perspective that helps you navigate through difficult times with grace and a positive mindset.

Shift from Comparison: Practicing gratitude helps you shift away from comparing yourself to others. Instead of focusing on what you lack, gratitude allows you to appreciate what you have, fostering self-acceptance and a healthier self-image, which contributes to a more youthful and confident demeanor.

Increased Energy: Gratitude can boost your energy levels. When you're grateful for the opportunities, experiences, and relationships in your life, it fuels your motivation and enthusiasm, making you feel more energized and ready to embrace life's adventures.

Ageless Joy: Gratitude reminds you to find joy in the present moment, regardless of age. It helps you maintain a childlike sense of wonder, curiosity, and appreciation for life's simple pleasures, creating a youthful and joyous spirit.

Be reminded, practicing gratitude is about incorporating a daily habit of acknowledging and expressing thanks for the blessings in your life. It's a mindset that can be cultivated through practices like journaling, expressing appreciation to others, or simply taking a moment each day to reflect on what you're grateful for. So, embrace the power of gratitude and infuse your life with youthful appreciation and positivity!

Chapter Fourteen

LIMIT ALCOHOL, TOBACCO, SMOKING AND HARD DRUGS CONSUMPTION

Limiting alcohol consumption, avoiding tobacco and smoking, and staying away from hard drugs can significantly contribute to promoting a youthful age. Here's a casual explanation of how these choices can benefit your overall well-being:

Healthier Body: Avoiding excessive alcohol consumption, tobacco, smoking, and hard drugs helps protect your body from the harmful effects associated with these substances. It reduces the risk of developing various health conditions, allowing your body to function optimally and maintain a youthful vitality.

Youthful Appearance: Alcohol, tobacco, smoking, and hard drugs can have negative effects on your physical appearance. They can contribute to premature aging, including wrinkles, dull skin, stained teeth, and other visible signs of damage. By limiting or avoiding these substances, you can maintain a more youthful and vibrant appearance.

Increased Energy: Substance abuse, such as excessive alcohol consumption and drug use, can drain your energy and leave you feeling lethargic. By limiting these substances, you can improve your energy levels, promoting a more youthful and active lifestyle.

Mental Clarity: Alcohol, tobacco, smoking, and hard drugs can impair cognitive function, memory, and overall mental clarity. By avoiding or limiting their use, you can enhance your mental focus, concentration, and decision-making abilities, fostering a sharper and more youthful mind.

Emotional Well-being: Substance abuse can negatively impact your emotional well-being, leading to mood swings, anxiety, and depression. By avoiding or moderating the use of alcohol, tobacco, smoking, and hard drugs, you can maintain a more stable and positive emotional state, contributing to a youthful and balanced outlook on life.

Enhanced Relationships: Substance abuse can strain relationships with friends, family, and loved ones. By making the choice to limit or avoid these substances, you can foster healthier and more meaningful connections, creating a positive and supportive social network that contributes to a more youthful and fulfilling life.

Longevity and Vitality: Alcohol abuse, tobacco, smoking, and hard drugs are associated with various health risks and can shorten your lifespan. By making healthier choices, you increase your chances of living a longer, more vibrant life, allowing you to enjoy a youthful age with vitality and vigor.

Personal Growth: Limiting or avoiding substances that impair judgment and decision-making enables personal growth and self-development. It allows you to make better choices, pursue meaningful goals, and invest in activities that contribute to your overall well-being, promoting a sense of personal fulfillment and a youthful sense of purpose.

Positive Role Modeling: By choosing to limit alcohol, tobacco, smoking, and hard drugs, you become a positive role model for others, especially younger individuals. Your actions can inspire them to make healthier choices, promoting a collective youthful mindset and a culture of well-being.

Freedom and Independence: By freeing yourself from the grip of alcohol, tobacco, smoking, and hard drugs, you reclaim your independence and control over your life. You become the master of your own destiny, making choices that align with your values and aspirations, leading to a more empowered and youthful existence.

Remember, embracing a lifestyle that limits or avoids these substances is a personal choice and can positively impact your overall well-being. It's about prioritizing your health, well-being, and embracing the possibilities that come with a youthful and substance-free life.

Chapter Fifteen

EMBRACE A POSITIVE MINDSET

Embracing a positive mindset can greatly contribute to promoting a youthful age. Here's an explanation of how a positive mindset can have a trans-formative effect:

Optimistic Outlook: A positive mindset involves adopting an optimistic outlook on life. It means focusing on possibilities, solutions, and the bright side of situations. By cultivating optimism, you can approach challenges with resilience and maintain a youthful and hopeful perspective.

Emotional Well-being: A positive mindset fosters emotional well-being. It involves managing negative emotions effectively and cultivating positive ones like joy, gratitude, and contentment. This emotional balance contributes to a more youthful and vibrant state of mind.

Stress Reduction: Embracing a positive mindset helps reduce stress. It involves re-framing negative thoughts, practicing self-care, and adopting coping mechanisms that promote relaxation and calmness. By managing stress effectively, you can prevent its negative impact on your overall well-being, keeping you youthful and energized.

Growth and Learning: A positive mindset encourages growth and learning. It involves embracing challenges as opportunities for personal development, seeking new experiences, and expanding your knowledge and skills. By embracing a mindset of continuous growth, you remain curious, adaptable, and open-minded, keeping your mind youthful and engaged.

Resilience and Adaptability: A positive mindset cultivates resilience and adaptability. It means bouncing back from setbacks, learning from failures, and finding opportunities for growth in difficult situations. By embracing resilience and adaptability, you maintain a youthful spirit that is undeterred by obstacles.

Self-Confidence: A positive mindset nurtures self-confidence. It involves recognizing your strengths, celebrating achievements, and believing in your abilities. With self-confidence, you approach life's challenges with a youthful determination and a belief that you can overcome them.

Healthy Relationships: A positive mindset fosters healthy relationships. It involves practicing empathy, kindness, and forgiveness towards others. By nurturing positive connections and surrounding yourself with supportive people, you create a social environment that promotes a youthful sense of belonging and happiness.

Energy and Vitality: A positive mindset boosts energy and vitality. It involves focusing on positive thoughts, engaging in activities that bring joy, and practicing self-care that replenishes your energy reserves. By maintaining high energy levels, you can approach life with enthusiasm and a youthful zest.

Gratitude and Appreciation: A positive mindset embraces gratitude and appreciation. It involves recognizing and expressing thanks for the blessings in your life, fostering a sense of abundance and contentment. By cultivating gratitude, you cultivate a youthful sense of wonder, joy, and appreciation for life's simple pleasures.

Youthful Perspective: A positive mindset maintains a youthful perspective on life. It involves embracing a sense of playfulness, curiosity, and wonder. By seeing the world through fresh eyes, you can tap into the vibrancy and enthusiasm that characterize youth.

Recall, developing a positive mindset is a journey that requires practice and self-awareness. It's about consciously choosing thoughts, beliefs, and attitudes that support your well-being and contribute to a youthful outlook. By embracing a positive mindset, you can navigate life's ups and downs with resilience, grace, and an unwavering youthful spirit.

Chapter Sixteen

STAY CURIOUS AND LEARN

Staying curious and embracing a love for learning can greatly promote a youthful age. Here's a brief explanation of how curiosity and learning contribute to maintaining a youthful mindset:

Intellectual Stimulation: Staying curious and seeking opportunities to learn keeps your mind active and engaged. It stimulates intellectual growth, preventing mental stagnation and promoting a youthful and agile mind.

Continuous Personal Growth: Embracing a love for learning means committing to ongoing personal growth. It involves seeking new knowledge, acquiring new skills, and expanding your understanding of the world. By pursuing personal growth, you maintain a sense of vitality and a youthful spirit of exploration.

Adaptability and Resilience: Curiosity and learning foster adaptability and resilience. They encourage you to embrace change, learn from experiences, and approach challenges with an open mind. By being adaptable and resilient, you navigate life's transitions with grace, maintaining a youthful and flexible outlook.

Creativity and Innovation: Curiosity fuels creativity and innovation. It prompts you to explore new ideas, think outside the box, and find unique solutions to problems. By nurturing your creative abilities, you tap into a wellspring of imagination and maintain a youthful and inventive approach to life.

Broadened Perspectives: Learning fosters empathy and broadens your perspectives. It exposes you to diverse cultures, ideas, and experiences, enhancing your understanding of the world. By embracing different perspectives, you cultivate a youthful curiosity and appreciation for the richness of human existence.

Sense of Wonder: Curiosity ignites a sense of wonder and awe. It encourages you to marvel at the mysteries of the world and find joy in the little things. By nurturing a sense of wonder, you maintain a youthful and enthusiastic appreciation for the beauty and magic of life.

Lifelong Learning: Embracing a love for learning means adopting a mindset of lifelong learning. It recognizes that learning is not limited to formal education but can occur in various aspects of life. By embracing the journey of continuous learning, you keep your mind open, adaptable, and youthful.

Personal Fulfillment: Curiosity and learning lead to personal fulfillment. They allow you to pursue interests, passions, and hobbies that bring you joy. By engaging in activities that ignite your curiosity, you cultivate a sense of purpose and fulfillment, contributing to a youthful and meaningful existence.

Enhanced Problem-Solving Skills: Learning nurtures problem-solving skills. It equips you with knowledge and critical thinking abilities to overcome challenges and find innovative solutions. By honing your problem-solving skills, you approach life's obstacles with a youthful and determined mindset.

Active Engagement with Life: Curiosity and learning keep you actively engaged with life. They inspire you to explore, discover, and seek new experiences. By staying curious and embracing a love for learning, you cultivate a zest for life that is inherently youthful and full of possibilities.

Recall, curiosity and learning are lifelong pursuits that can be embraced in various ways. Whether through reading, exploring new hobbies, traveling, or engaging in conversations with others, staying curious allows you to continue growing, discovering, and maintaining a youthful and vibrant perspective on the world.

Chapter Seventeen

PRACTICING MINDFUL AGING

Practicing mindful aging can promote a youthful age by cultivating a positive and present-focused mindset. Here's an explanation of how mindful aging contributes to maintaining a youthful outlook:

Living in the Present: Mindful aging encourages you to live in the present moment, appreciating and fully experiencing each stage of life. By focusing on the here and now, you can let go of regrets about the past and worries about the future, fostering a sense of youthfulness and contentment.

Acceptance and Self-Compassion: Mindful aging involves accepting yourself and embracing self-compassion. It means acknowledging the changes that come with age and being kind to yourself through the process. By practicing self-acceptance and self-compassion, you can maintain a positive self-image and a youthful sense of self-worth.

Gratitude for Aging: Mindful aging cultivates gratitude for the aging process itself. It involves appreciating the wisdom, experiences, and opportunities that come with getting older. By expressing gratitude for the journey of aging, you foster a sense of appreciation and a youthful perspective on the value of each passing year.

Emotional Resilience: Mindful aging enhances emotional resilience. It equips you with tools to navigate the challenges that may arise with aging, such as health changes or life transitions. By cultivating emotional resilience, you can adapt to changes with grace and maintain a youthful spirit of resilience and optimism.

Mind-Body Connection: Mindful aging recognizes the interconnectedness of the mind and body. It involves nourishing both aspects through practices such as meditation, mindful movement, and self-care. By nurturing the mind-body connection, you promote vitality and a youthful sense of overall well-being.

Healthy Lifestyle Choices: Mindful aging encourages making healthy lifestyle choices. It involves being conscious of nutrition, exercise, and self-care habits that support optimal well-being. By prioritizing health and well-being, you can maintain physical vitality and a youthful energy that transcends age.

Meaningful Relationships: Mindful aging fosters meaningful connections and relationships. It involves investing time and energy into nurturing relationships with loved ones, building a supportive social network, and creating a sense of belonging. By cultivating meaningful relationships, you foster a youthful sense of connection, joy, and companionship.

Continued Growth and Learning: Mindful aging embraces a mindset of continued growth and learning. It involves seeking new experiences, acquiring knowledge, and engaging in activities that expand your horizons. By pursuing growth and learning, you keep your mind active, curious, and youthful.

Letting Go of Attachments: Mindful aging encourages letting go of attachments to societal expectations, past identities, or material possessions. It involves embracing the freedom that comes with releasing what no longer serves you. By letting go, you create space for new possibilities, growth, and a youthful sense of liberation.

Embracing Transitions: Mindful aging involves embracing life transitions with openness and grace. It recognizes that change is a natural part of the human experience and that each transition brings opportunities for growth and renewal. By embracing transitions, you maintain a sense of excitement, adaptability, and a youthful outlook on life's ever-evolving journey.

Remember, practicing mindful aging is a personal journey that involves cultivating awareness, acceptance, and gratitude for each moment. By embracing the present, nurturing your well-being, and fostering meaningful connections, you can maintain a youthful perspective and age with grace, wisdom, and a vibrant spirit.

Chapter Eighteen

EXPRESS YOURSELF

Expressing yourself can promote a youthful age by fostering a sense of authenticity, creativity, and personal growth. Here's a casual explanation of how expressing yourself contributes to maintaining a youthful outlook:

Authenticity: Expressing yourself allows you to embrace and showcase your true self. It involves being genuine, honest, and unafraid to show your unique personality, preferences, and opinions. By embracing authenticity, you cultivate a sense of self-confidence and a youthful spirit that celebrates individuality.

Self-Discovery: Expressing yourself encourages self-discovery and self-awareness. It involves exploring your passions, interests, and talents, and allowing them to shine. By engaging in activities that align with your true self, you uncover new aspects of your identity, fostering personal growth and a youthful sense of curiosity.

Creativity and Innovation: Expressing yourself nurtures creativity and innovation. It means finding unique ways to express your thoughts, emotions, and ideas through art, writing, music, or any other form of creative expression. By tapping into your creative potential, you maintain a youthful and imaginative perspective on life.

Emotional Well-being: Expressing yourself supports emotional well-being. It allows you to release and communicate your feelings, reducing emotional tension and promoting inner harmony. By expressing both positive and negative emotions constructively, you cultivate emotional resilience and a youthful sense of emotional balance.

Communication Skills: Expressing yourself hones your communication skills. It involves effectively articulating your thoughts, actively listening to others, and engaging in meaningful conversations. By developing strong communication skills, you foster positive connections with others, contributing to a youthful and vibrant social life.

Confidence and Self-Esteem: Expressing yourself boosts confidence and self-esteem. It involves speaking up, asserting yourself, and sharing your ideas and perspectives with others. By valuing your own voice and opinions, you maintain a youthful and empowered sense of self-worth.

Personal Empowerment: Expressing yourself empowers you to take ownership of your life. It means making choices that align with your values and desires, setting boundaries, and advocating for yourself. By embracing personal empowerment, you maintain a youthful and proactive approach to shaping your own destiny.

Problem-Solving and Innovation: Expressing yourself nurtures problem-solving and innovative thinking. It encourages you to find creative solutions, think outside the box, and embrace new ideas. By applying your unique perspective to challenges, you cultivate a youthful and resourceful mindset.

Connection and Relatability: Expressing yourself facilitates connection and relatability with others. It allows you to share experiences, stories, and passions, creating bonds and fostering a sense of community. By connecting with others authentically, you maintain a youthful and vibrant social network.

Personal Fulfillment: Expressing yourself leads to personal fulfillment. It means pursuing activities that bring you joy, satisfaction, and a sense of purpose. By expressing yourself in ways that resonate with your deepest desires, you cultivate a youthful and fulfilling life that is aligned with your authentic self.

Recall, expressing yourself is a lifelong journey of self-discovery and growth. Whether through art, writing, conversation, or any other form of self-expression, embracing and celebrating your unique voice contributes to maintaining a youthful spirit that embraces authenticity, creativity, and personal fulfillment.

Chapter Nineteen

STAY HYGENIC

Staying hygienic can promote a youthful age by preserving your health, enhancing your appearance, and boosting your overall well-being. Here's a simple explanation of how practicing good hygiene contributes to maintaining a youthful outlook:

Skin Health: Proper hygiene, such as regular cleansing and moisturizing, helps keep your skin clean and healthy. It removes dirt, oils, and impurities that can lead to skin issues like acne or dullness. By maintaining clean and well-moisturized skin, you promote a youthful and radiant complexion.

Oral Health: Maintaining good oral hygiene, including regular brushing, flossing, and dental check-ups, contributes to a youthful appearance. It prevents tooth decay, gum diseases, and bad breath, ensuring a healthy and attractive smile. By taking care of your oral health, you preserve a youthful and vibrant appearance.

Hair Care: Practicing proper hair hygiene, such as regular washing and conditioning, helps keep your hair clean, shiny, and healthy-looking. It prevents scalp issues, excessive oiliness, or dandruff that can affect the appearance of your hair. By maintaining clean and well-groomed hair, you exude a youthful and put-together image.

Personal Odor: Practicing good hygiene by regularly bathing or showering helps eliminate body odor, leaving you feeling fresh and confident. By maintaining personal cleanliness and using deodorants or antiperspirants, you ensure a pleasant scent, contributing to a youthful and pleasant presence.

Preventing Illness: Good hygiene habits, such as frequent hand-washing and sanitizing, help prevent the spread of germs and reduce the risk of infections and illnesses. By maintaining a healthy body and immune system, you can avoid the negative impacts that illnesses can have on your overall well-being and youthful vitality.

Confidence and Self-Esteem: Staying hygienic enhances your self-confidence and self-esteem. When you feel clean, fresh, and well-groomed, you project a positive image and feel good about yourself. By exuding confidence and self-assuredness, you radiate a youthful energy and attractiveness.

Social Interactions: Good hygiene promotes positive social interactions. When you maintain personal cleanliness and freshness, you create a comfortable environment for yourself and those around you. By presenting yourself well, you can engage in social interactions with ease, fostering meaningful connections and maintaining a youthful and vibrant social life.

Overall Well-being: Practicing good hygiene contributes to your overall well-being. It shows that you prioritize self-care and take responsibility for your health. By adopting hygienic practices, you can experience higher energy levels, improved mood, and a greater sense of vitality, all of which contribute to a youthful and positive outlook on life.

Professional Image: Maintaining good hygiene is important for your professional image. A clean and well-groomed appearance instills trust and professionalism. By presenting yourself in a polished manner, you project a youthful and capable image that can positively impact your career and personal growth.

Long-Term Health: Good hygiene habits have long-term benefits for your health. By preventing infections, diseases, and other health issues, you promote longevity and preserve your youthful vigor. By taking care of your body through proper hygiene, you invest in your long-term well-being.

Remember, good hygiene practices are simple yet powerful habits that can significantly contribute to your overall health, appearance, and well-being. By incorporating them into your daily routine, you can maintain a youthful and vibrant image while enjoying the numerous benefits of a hygienic lifestyle.

SUMMARY

To maintain a youthful age, here's a *SUMMARY* of key practices

Take care of your physical health by staying active, eating a balanced diet, staying hydrated, protecting your skin from the sun, getting enough sleep, and managing stress.

Engage in activities that bring you joy and laughter, have fun, and embrace a positive mindset.

Stay socially connected, nurture meaningful relationships, and surround yourself with supportive and like-minded individuals.

Prioritize self-care, including skincare routines, maintaining good posture, protecting your eyes, and practicing gratitude.

Avoid harmful substances such as alcohol, tobacco, smoking, and hard drugs.

Embrace a positive and curious mindset, challenge your mind, and continue learning throughout your life.

Practice mindfulness and embrace the aging process with acceptance, grace, and resilience.

Express yourself authentically, nurture your creativity, and seek personal fulfillment.

Practice good hygiene, including taking care of your skin, oral health, hair, and personal odor.

By incorporating these practices into your lifestyle, you can promote a youthful age by taking care of your physical, mental, and emotional well-being, maintaining positive outlook, and embracing a vibrant and fulfilling life.